Essential Oil Toolkit &

Recipe Journal

This Book Belongs to

_____

Dedicated to those whose lives have been
enriched by essential oils

Disclaimer

This book contains information to help support individuals with their use of essential oils. While I have made every attempt to verify that the information provided in this book is correct and up to date, I assume no responsibility for any error, inaccuracy, or omission.

The advice, recipes, and examples herein are not suitable for every situation. The materials contained herein are not intended to represent or guarantee that you will achieve your desired outcome, and I make no such guarantee. Results are determined by a number of factors beyond my control including, but not limited to, quality of essential oils, reader's accurate measurement when creating the recipes, body's tolerance of essential oils and medical conditions.

The statements in this publication have not been evaluated by the Food and Drug Administration. These products & recipes are not intended to diagnose, treat, cure, or prevent disease.

Table of Contents

How to use this book

My purpose for creating this book is to give you a quick guide to make living with essential oils easier! There are 2 different parts of this book, the first section is your tool kit to keep all important information and charts in one place. The second section holds a variety of recipes and tons of space for you to add your own! So lets get started!

Section I

Chapter 1 is your Essential Oil Toolkit! In this section you will find pages and charts to help you organize your life with essential oils (both personally or for your EO business). This includes:

1) Fill in Index

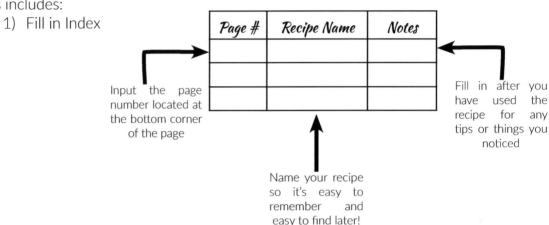

Page #	Recipe Name	Notes

Input the page number located at the bottom corner of the page

Fill in after you have used the recipe for any tips or things you noticed

Name your recipe so it's easy to remember and easy to find later!

2) Safety Guide including
   - Topical safety
   - Use with children
   - Photosensitive Oils
   - Dilution Chart & more!
3) A reflexology chart to help when applying essential oils to your feet
4) Inventory Checklist to keep track of all your oils
5) Colouring page - Just for fun!
6) List of who you have given samples to

Section 2

Section 2 is where you can record the essential oil recipes you have tried & want to make again or record recipes for future use. This section is broken into 4 chapters:

Chapter 2: Diffuser Recipes
Chapter 3: Roller Bottle Recipes
Chapter 4: DIY Essential Oil Recipes
Chapter 5: Essential Oil Cleaning Recipes

In each section you will find a few recipes that I have used and love that I thought you may like. There are also tons of empty recipe cards where you can record the ingredients needed, instructions & important usage notes!

Also to help you keep track of all of the recipes, you can record the recipe name, page number & other notes in your 'Fill in Index' found in your Toolkit. This will help you to easily find the recipe when you need it! You can find the index on page 14 and instructions on how to use it on the page to your left.

Here is an example of the recipe card

What You Need:

Title

How to make It:

Supplies needed

Note:

Instructions

What worked well, what didn't, any substitutions or what you used it for

Oil up Buttercup

Part 1: Essential Oil Tool Kit

Create your own Index

Keep track of the recipes you have added using this index page!

Page #	Recipe Name	Notes

Page #	Recipe Name	Notes

Page #	Recipe Name	Notes

Page #	Recipe Name	Notes

Essential Oil Safety Guide

Although essential oils have many benefits for naturally supporting health & wellness, it is important to know that they are VERY potent. Due to the potency levels it is extremely important that you are aware of essential oil safety tips and guidelines!

Essential Oil Safety for Topical Use

When using essential oils topically there are a number of important safety considerations that you should be aware of:

- Essential Oil Dilution
- Topical Essential Oil Use with Children
- Photosensitive Essential Oils

I will cover each of these areas in detail below!

Essential Oil Dilution

Using a carrier oil such as fractionated coconut oil, grapeseed oil or jojoba oil helps to dilute essential oils. There are a number of reasons to dilute your oils:

- Using Hot Oils
- Using Oils on a Large Area of Skin
- Photosensitive Oils
- Using Oils on Children

All of these reasons are covered in the sections below.

Diluting Hot Oils

There are a number of oils that are considered 'hot oils'. If you use these essential oils topically without diluting them first, they will actually cause a physical burn on your skin. When you are using hot essential oils you want to dilute them to 0.5% this means 1 drop for every 2 teaspoons of carrier oil. I recommend storing the diluted oil in a roller bottle (for easy application) or you could recycle an empty essential oil bottle. This is not an exhaustive list of 'hot oils' but does include some of the more popular ones.

Common 'HOT OILS' Include:

- Cassia
- Cinnamon
- Clove
- Cumin
- Oregano
- Thyme

Using Essential Oils on a Large Area of Skin

If you are wanting to use essential oils across a larger area such as your shoulders or back, it is important that you use a carrier oil to help the oils spread further. Adding more essential oil to cover the space is not a wise idea. Instead, mix the essential oil with a carrier oil. A common dilution ratio for this type of use is 3% meaning you want to mix 3 drops of essential oil with 1 teaspoon of carrier oil.

Photosensitive Essential Oils

Some oils are light-sensitive which means you should avoid direct sunlight for 12-24 hours when using them. To get around this, I will often apply the oils to my feet and then put on a pair of socks. If these oils are exposed to direct sunlight they could cause you to develop a burn on your skin. This is not an exhaustive list of 'Photosensitive Oils' but does include some of the more popular ones.

Photosensitive oils include:
- Bergamot
- Grapefruit
- Lemon
- Lime

Additional Safety Tips of Topical Use of Essential Oils

Keep oils away from your eyes!

After using oils make sure to wash your hands thoroughly. Learn from my mistakes, I have on more than one occasion not washed my hands immediately after applying oils and then out of habit rubbed my eyes.... It is a very, very uncomfortable feeling!

Tip: If you get essential oils in/near your eye:
1. Wash your hands thoroughly with soap
2. Apply fractionated coconut oil around the outside of your closed eye- this will help take the pain away in less than 30 seconds.

Topical Use with Children

Before jumping into how to use essential oils with children, let's first discuss which oils are generally safe for children of different ages. Please note that this is not an exhaustive list but does include the more popular/ commonly used essential oils.

When using essential oils with children under 2, I recommend that you always consult with a medical professional and/or certified aromatherapist prior to use.

The following information is based off of Tisserand & Young's Essential Oil Safety Textbook. This chart refers to essential oils in general and is not based on any specific brand of essential oils.

The following oils are NOT SAFE to use with children under 2

Anise	Lemongrass
Basil	Marjoram
Bay (Laurel)	May Chang (Litsea Cubeba)
Birch	Melissa
Cajeput	Myrtle (all)
Camphor	Opopanax
Cardamom	Oregano
Cassia	Peppermint
Cedarwood (Himalayan)	Ravintsara
Clove Bud	Rosemary
Eucalyptus	Sage
Fennel	Wintergreen
Garlic	Ylang Ylang

The following oils are NOT SAFE for children under 5

Anise	Myrtle (aniseed, red)
Bay (Laurel)	Opopanax
Birch	Peppermint
Cajeput	Ravintsara
Camphor	Rosemary
Cardamom	Sage
Eucalyptus	Wintergreen
Marjoram	

If you are using essential oils with children it is extremely important that you dilute the oils. The potency level undiluted is too strong for children.

For children age 6 months to 6 years you want to use a 0.5% dilution ratio. This means 2 teaspoons of carrier oil for every 1 drop of essential oil.

With children over age 6 mix 1 drop of essential oil with 1 teaspoon of essential oil.

Essential oil safety tip for topical use with children: I recommend either applying the diluted oils to your child's feet and cover with socks or apply to their chest (i.e. when use is for congestion) and then cover with a sleeper or undershirt. This will help to ensure that your child doesn't get the oils on their hands and rub it in their eyes.

Essential Oil Dilution Ratios & How to Create Them

Understanding dilution ratios can be quite confusing! Keep this chart close by to help you easily dilute your favourite oils & create blends.

Dilution Ratio	How to Make It	Recommended for
0.5%	1 drop essential oil per 2 teaspoons of carrier oil	• Diluting 'hot oils' • For use with children 6 months to 6 years of age. Always consult with a medical professional for use with children under 2 years of age.
1%	1 drop essential oil per every teaspoon of carrier oil or 5-6 drops per ounce	• For use in children over the age of 6 • Elderly adults • Pregnant women (ensure oil is safe to use during pregnancy) • Those with preexisting health conditions.
2%	2 drops essential oil per teaspoon of carrier oil or 10-12 drops per ounce	• For use with most adults.
3%	3 drops essential oil per teaspoon of carrier oil or 15-18 drops per ounce	• For use with most adults.

Reflexology Chart

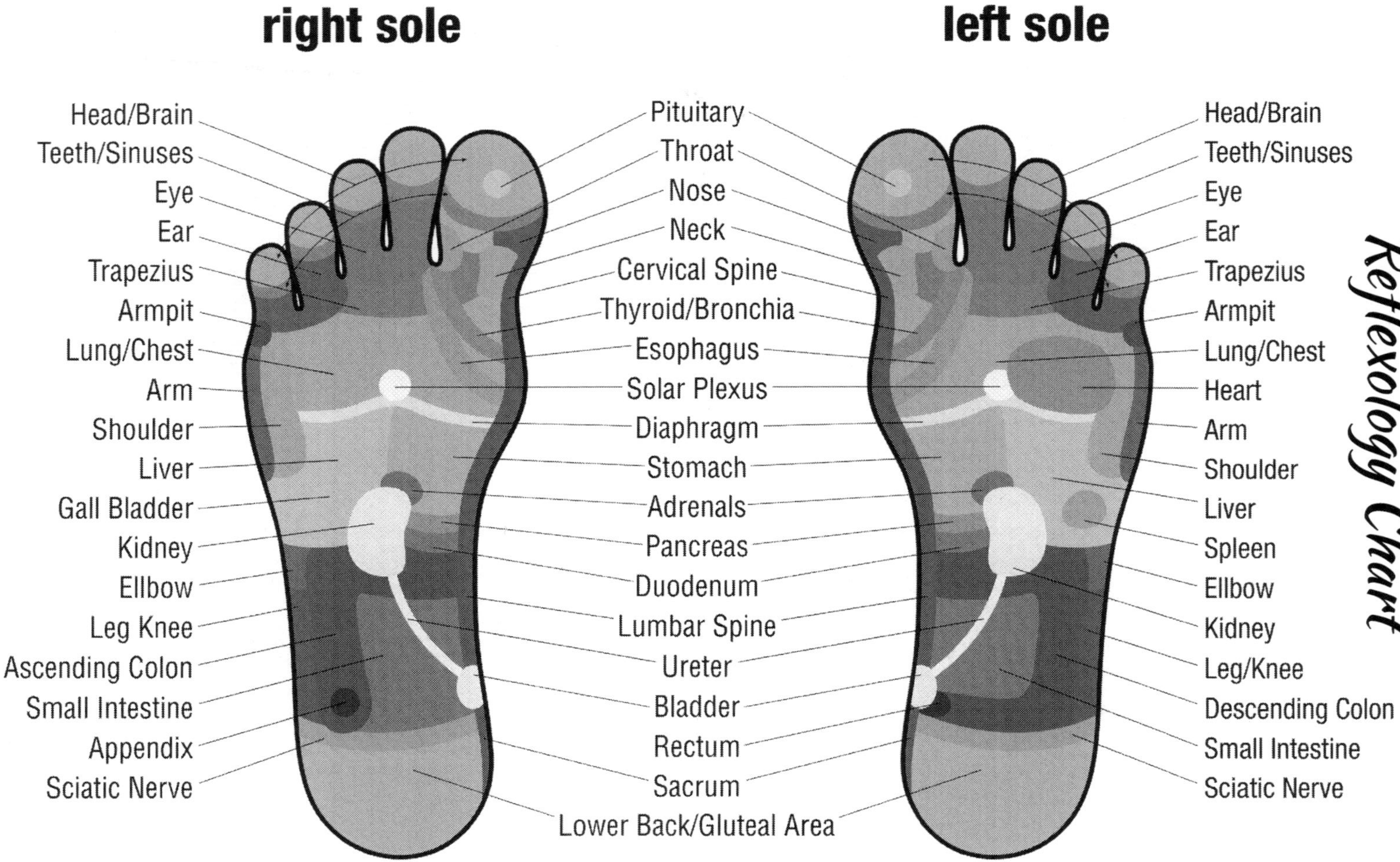

left sole

right sole

left sole labels:
Head/Brain
Teeth/Sinuses
Eye
Ear
Trapezius
Armpit
Lung/Chest
Heart
Arm
Shoulder
Liver
Spleen
Ellbow
Kidney
Leg/Knee
Descending Colon
Small Intestine
Sciatic Nerve

Pituitary
Throat
Nose
Neck
Cervical Spine
Thyroid/Bronchia
Esophagus
Solar Plexus
Diaphragm
Stomach
Adrenals
Pancreas
Duodenum
Lumbar Spine
Ureter
Bladder
Rectum
Sacrum
Lower Back/Gluteal Area

right sole labels:
Head/Brain
Teeth/Sinuses
Eye
Ear
Trapezius
Armpit
Lung/Chest
Arm
Shoulder
Liver
Gall Bladder
Kidney
Ellbow
Leg Knee
Ascending Colon
Small Intestine
Appendix
Sciatic Nerve

medial side of both feet

lateral side of both feet

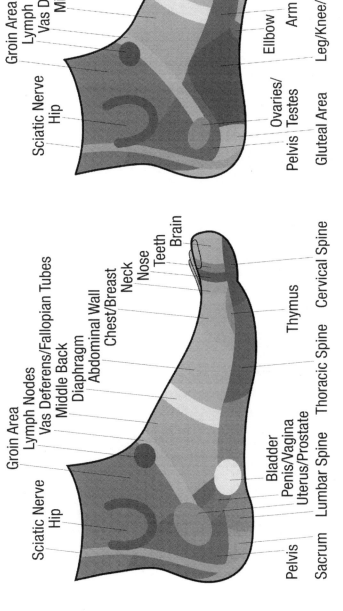

medial side of both feet labels:
- Sciatic Nerve
- Hip
- Groin Area
- Lymph Nodes
- Vas Deferens/Fallopian Tubes
- Middle Back
- Diaphragm
- Abdominal Wall
- Chest/Breast
- Neck
- Nose
- Teeth
- Brain
- Cervical Spine
- Thoracic Spine
- Thymus
- Lumbar Spine
- Bladder
- Penis/Vagina
- Uterus/Prostate
- Sacrum
- Pelvis

lateral side of both feet labels:
- Groin Area
- Lymph Nodes
- Vas Deferens/Fallopian Tubes
- Middle Back
- Diaphragm
- Abdominal Wall
- Chest/Breast
- Head
- Sciatic Nerve
- Hip
- Ear
- Leg/Knee/Lower Back
- Shoulder
- Arm
- Elbow
- Ovaries/Testes
- Pelvis
- Gluteal Area

Oily Inventory

Oil	1st Bottle					2nd Bottle					Wish List
	Buy	1/4	1/2	3/4	Full	Buy	1/4	1/2	3/4	Full	
ARBORVITAE	○	○	○	○	○	○	○	○	○	○	○
BALSAM FIR	○	○	○	○	○	○	○	○	○	○	○
BASIL	○	○	○	○	○	○	○	○	○	○	○
BERGAMOT	○	○	○	○	○	○	○	○	○	○	○
BLACK PEPPER	○	○	○	○	○	○	○	○	○	○	○
CARDAMOM	○	○	○	○	○	○	○	○	○	○	○
CASSIA	○	○	○	○	○	○	○	○	○	○	○
CEDARWOOD	○	○	○	○	○	○	○	○	○	○	○
CILANTRO	○	○	○	○	○	○	○	○	○	○	○
CINNAMON BARK	○	○	○	○	○	○	○	○	○	○	○
CLARY SAGE	○	○	○	○	○	○	○	○	○	○	○
CLOVE	○	○	○	○	○	○	○	○	○	○	○
COPAIBA	○	○	○	○	○	○	○	○	○	○	○
CORIANDER	○	○	○	○	○	○	○	○	○	○	○
CUMIN	○	○	○	○	○	○	○	○	○	○	○
CYPRESS	○	○	○	○	○	○	○	○	○	○	○
DILL	○	○	○	○	○	○	○	○	○	○	○
DOUGLAS FIR	○	○	○	○	○	○	○	○	○	○	○
EUCALYPTUS	○	○	○	○	○	○	○	○	○	○	○
FRANKINCENSE	○	○	○	○	○	○	○	○	○	○	○
FENNEL	○	○	○	○	○	○	○	○	○	○	○
GERANIUM	○	○	○	○	○	○	○	○	○	○	○
GINGER	○	○	○	○	○	○	○	○	○	○	○
GRAPEFRUIT	○	○	○	○	○	○	○	○	○	○	○
HELICHRYSUM	○	○	○	○	○	○	○	○	○	○	○
JASMINE	○	○	○	○	○	○	○	○	○	○	○
JUNIPER	○	○	○	○	○	○	○	○	○	○	○
LAVENDER	○	○	○	○	○	○	○	○	○	○	○

Oil	1st Bottle					2nd Bottle					Wish List
	Buy	1/4	1/2	3/4	Full	Buy	1/4	1/2	3/4	Full	
LEMON	○	○	○	○	○	○	○	○	○	○	○
LEMONGRASS	○	○	○	○	○	○	○	○	○	○	○
LIME	○	○	○	○	○	○	○	○	○	○	○
MARJORAM	○	○	○	○	○	○	○	○	○	○	○
MELALEUCA/TEA TREE	○	○	○	○	○	○	○	○	○	○	○
MELISSA	○	○	○	○	○	○	○	○	○	○	○
MYRRH	○	○	○	○	○	○	○	○	○	○	○
NEROLI	○	○	○	○	○	○	○	○	○	○	○
OREGANO	○	○	○	○	○	○	○	○	○	○	○
PATCHOULI	○	○	○	○	○	○	○	○	○	○	○
PEPPERMINT	○	○	○	○	○	○	○	○	○	○	○
PETITGRAIN	○	○	○	○	○	○	○	○	○	○	○
PINE	○	○	○	○	○	○	○	○	○	○	○
ROMAN CHAMOMILE	○	○	○	○	○	○	○	○	○	○	○
ROSE	○	○	○	○	○	○	○	○	○	○	○
ROSEMARY	○	○	○	○	○	○	○	○	○	○	○
SAGE	○	○	○	○	○	○	○	○	○	○	○
SANDALWOOD (HAWAIIAN)	○	○	○	○	○	○	○	○	○	○	○
SANDALWOOD (INDIAN)	○	○	○	○	○	○	○	○	○	○	○
SPEARMINT	○	○	○	○	○	○	○	○	○	○	○
SPIKENARD	○	○	○	○	○	○	○	○	○	○	○
TANGERINE	○	○	○	○	○	○	○	○	○	○	○
THYME	○	○	○	○	○	○	○	○	○	○	○
VETIVER	○	○	○	○	○	○	○	○	○	○	○
WHITE FIR	○	○	○	○	○	○	○	○	○	○	○
WILD ORANGE	○	○	○	○	○	○	○	○	○	○	○
WINTERGREEN	○	○	○	○	○	○	○	○	○	○	○
YLANG YLANG	○	○	○	○	○	○	○	○	○	○	○

| Oil | 1st Bottle | | | | | 2nd Bottle | | | | | Wish List |
Fill in your Own	Buy	1/4	1/2	3/4	Full	Buy	1/4	1/2	3/4	Full	
_____	◯	◯	◯	◯	◯	◯	◯	◯	◯	◯	◯
_____	◯	◯	◯	◯	◯	◯	◯	◯	◯	◯	◯
_____	◯	◯	◯	◯	◯	◯	◯	◯	◯	◯	◯
_____	◯	◯	◯	◯	◯	◯	◯	◯	◯	◯	◯
_____	◯	◯	◯	◯	◯	◯	◯	◯	◯	◯	◯
_____	◯	◯	◯	◯	◯	◯	◯	◯	◯	◯	◯
_____	◯	◯	◯	◯	◯	◯	◯	◯	◯	◯	◯
_____	◯	◯	◯	◯	◯	◯	◯	◯	◯	◯	◯
_____	◯	◯	◯	◯	◯	◯	◯	◯	◯	◯	◯
_____	◯	◯	◯	◯	◯	◯	◯	◯	◯	◯	◯
_____	◯	◯	◯	◯	◯	◯	◯	◯	◯	◯	◯
_____	◯	◯	◯	◯	◯	◯	◯	◯	◯	◯	◯
_____	◯	◯	◯	◯	◯	◯	◯	◯	◯	◯	◯
_____	◯	◯	◯	◯	◯	◯	◯	◯	◯	◯	◯
_____	◯	◯	◯	◯	◯	◯	◯	◯	◯	◯	◯
_____	◯	◯	◯	◯	◯	◯	◯	◯	◯	◯	◯
_____	◯	◯	◯	◯	◯	◯	◯	◯	◯	◯	◯
_____	◯	◯	◯	◯	◯	◯	◯	◯	◯	◯	◯
_____	◯	◯	◯	◯	◯	◯	◯	◯	◯	◯	◯
_____	◯	◯	◯	◯	◯	◯	◯	◯	◯	◯	◯
_____	◯	◯	◯	◯	◯	◯	◯	◯	◯	◯	◯

Oil	1st Bottle					2nd Bottle					Wish List
Blends	Buy	1/4	1/2	3/4	Full	Buy	1/4	1/2	3/4	Full	
_____	○	○	○	○	○	○	○	○	○	○	○
_____	○	○	○	○	○	○	○	○	○	○	○
_____	○	○	○	○	○	○	○	○	○	○	○
_____	○	○	○	○	○	○	○	○	○	○	○
_____	○	○	○	○	○	○	○	○	○	○	○
_____	○	○	○	○	○	○	○	○	○	○	○
_____	○	○	○	○	○	○	○	○	○	○	○
_____	○	○	○	○	○	○	○	○	○	○	○
_____	○	○	○	○	○	○	○	○	○	○	○
_____	○	○	○	○	○	○	○	○	○	○	○
_____	○	○	○	○	○	○	○	○	○	○	○
_____	○	○	○	○	○	○	○	○	○	○	○
_____	○	○	○	○	○	○	○	○	○	○	○
_____	○	○	○	○	○	○	○	○	○	○	○
_____	○	○	○	○	○	○	○	○	○	○	○
_____	○	○	○	○	○	○	○	○	○	○	○
_____	○	○	○	○	○	○	○	○	○	○	○
_____	○	○	○	○	○	○	○	○	○	○	○
_____	○	○	○	○	○	○	○	○	○	○	○
_____	○	○	○	○	○	○	○	○	○	○	○
_____	○	○	○	○	○	○	○	○	○	○	○

Tracking Samples

Use this sheet to keep track of the samples you have given, who you gave them to and their contact information so you can follow up!

Date	Name	Oil Given	Follow Up Info	Follow Up Done?

Date	Name	Oil Given	Follow Up Info	Follow Up Done?

Date	Name	Oil Given	Follow Up Info	Follow Up Done?

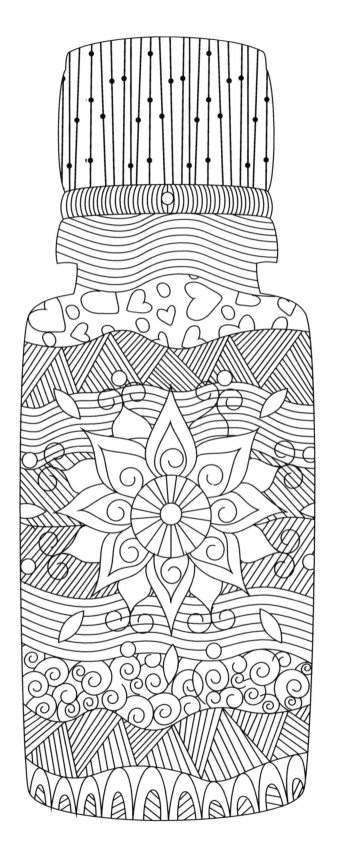

If you love someone, give them essential oils!

Part 2: Diffuser Recipes

Mid-Afternoon Pick Me Up

What You Need:

2 drops peppermint

2 drops lime

How to Make It:

1) Simply add the oils to the water in your diffuser (following your diffuser's manual).

Note:

This recipe is meant for diffusers that hold a minimum of 200ml of water. If you have a smaller diffuser you will want to use fewer oils.

Since this recipe uses peppermint I would not recommend using it before bed.

Changing Seasons Tickle My Nose

What You Need:

1-2 drops of lemon

1-2 drops of peppermint

1-2 drops of lavender

How to Make It:

1) Simply add the oils to the water in your diffuser (following your diffuser's manual).

Note:

For diffusers under 200ml use 1 drop of each oil, for larger diffusers you can use 2 drops of each. If you get congested, have runny eyes and a headache during seasonal changes then this recipe may be just what you need to feel better!

Spring Cleaning

What You Need:

4 drops lime

2 drops wild orange

How to Make It:

1) Simply add the oils to the water in your diffuser (following your

diffuser's manual).

Note:

For diffusers under 200ml use 1 drop of each oil, for larger diffusers you

can use 2 drops of each. This blend removes stale air when diffused and

is a wonderful microbial when used in the kitchen.

Another Rainy Day

What You Need:

2 drops vetiver

1 drop lemon

1 drop lavender

How to Make It:

1) Simply add the oils to the water in your diffuser (following your

diffuser's manual).

Note:

For diffusers under 200ml use 1 drop of each oil, for larger diffusers you

can use 2 drops of each.

What You Need:

_____   _____

_____   _____

How to make It:

_____

_____

Note:

_____

_____

What You Need:

_____   _____

_____   _____

How to make It:

_____

_____

Note:

_____

_____

What You Need:

_____   _____

_____   _____

How to make It:

_____

_____

Note:

_____

_____

_____

What You Need:

_____   _____

_____   _____

How to make It:

_____

_____

Note:

_____

_____

What You Need:

_____   _____

_____   _____

How to make It:

_____

_____

Note:

_____

_____

What You Need:

_____   _____

_____   _____

How to make It:

_____

_____

Note:

_____

_____

What You Need:

_____ _____

_____ _____

How to make It:

_____

_____

Note:

_____

_____

What You Need:

_____ _____

_____ _____

How to make It:

_____

_____

Note:

_____

_____

What You Need:

_____   _____

_____   _____

How to make It:

_____

_____

Note:

_____

_____

_____

What You Need:

_____   _____

_____   _____

How to make It:

_____

_____

Note:

_____

_____

What You Need:

_____   _____
_____   _____

How to make It:

_____
_____

Note:

_____
_____

What You Need:

_____   _____
_____   _____

How to make It:

_____
_____

Note:

_____
_____

What You Need:

_____   _____

_____   _____

How to make It:

_____

_____

Note:

_____

_____

_____

What You Need:

_____   _____

_____   _____

How to make It:

_____

_____

Note:

_____

_____

What You Need:

_____ _____

_____ _____

How to make It:

_____

_____

Note:

_____

_____

What You Need:

_____ _____

_____ _____

How to make It:

_____

_____

Note:

_____

_____

What You Need:

_____   _____

_____   _____

How to make It:

_____

_____

Note:

_____

_____

What You Need:

_____   _____

_____   _____

How to make It:

_____

_____

Note:

_____

_____

What You Need:

_____   _____

_____   _____

How to make It:

_____

_____

Note:

_____

_____

_____

What You Need:

_____   _____

_____   _____

How to make It:

_____

_____

Note:

_____

_____

What You Need:

_____   _____

_____   _____

How to make It:

_____

_____

Note:

_____

_____

What You Need:

_____   _____

_____   _____

How to make It:

_____

_____

Note:

_____

_____

What You Need:

_____   _____

_____   _____

How to make It:

_____

_____

Note:

_____

_____

_____

What You Need:

_____   _____

_____   _____

How to make It:

_____

_____

Note:

_____

_____

What You Need:

_____   _____

_____   _____

How to make It:

_____

_____

Note:

_____

_____

What You Need:

_____   _____

_____   _____

How to make It:

_____

_____

Note:

_____

_____

What You Need:

_____   _____

_____   _____

How to make It:

_____

_____

Note:

_____

_____

What You Need:

_____   _____

_____   _____

How to make It:

_____

_____

Note:

_____

_____

What You Need:

_____   _____

_____   _____

How to make It:

_____

_____

Note:

_____

_____

What You Need:

_____   _____

_____   _____

How to make It:

_____

_____

Note:

_____

_____

What You Need:

_____   _____

_____   _____

How to make It:

_____

_____

Note:

_____

_____

_____

What You Need:

_____   _____

_____   _____

How to make It:

_____

_____

Note:

_____

_____

"I simply can't think of another Essential Oil that I want to add to my collection."

-Said no one ever

Part 3: Roller Ball Recipes

Stress Be Gone

18+

What You Need:

3 drops Lavender

3 drops Frankincense

1 drop melissa

How to Make It:

1) Add oils to a 10ml roller bottle and fill to the top with a carrier oil such as fractionated coconut oil. Shake bottle before each use.

2) Apply to inside of wrists & back of neck. Alternatively I will do a swipe on the bottom of each foot.

Note:

This recipe is a 3.5% dilution ratio. If you don't have melissa simply skip it and the it will be 3% dilution. You can adjust this recipe to best suit your needs, see the dilution chart on page 21. Recipe is meant for adults.

Pain in the...

18+

What You Need:

2 drops White Fir

2 drops Lemongrass

2 drops Wintergreen

How to Make It:

1) Add oils to a 10ml roller bottle and fill to the top with a carrier oil such as fractionated coconut oil. Shake bottle before each use.

2) Apply this blend to the area that is causing you pain. It is great for sore muscles & joints.

Note:

This recipe has a 3% dilution ratio. You may want to adjust it based on your needs, see the dilution chart on page 21. Recipe is meant for adults.

Sleep, congestion and upset tummy

2+

What You Need:

2 drops of Lavender

How to Make It:

1) Add oils to a 10ml roller bottle and fill to the top with a carrier oil such as fractionated coconut oil. Shake bottle before each use.

2) Apply a short swipe on the bottoms of their feet.

Note:

This recipe is VERY simple and one that has multiple uses for little ones. This recipe is a 1% dilution ratio. Safety note: ALWAYS test on a small patch of skin when you are introducing new oils to see if your child has any reaction. Apply oils to bottom of feet (covered with socks) to help ensure that they don't rub any in their eyes. Consult with a medical professional prior to use.

Dreamland

18+

What You Need:

3 drops of Bergamot   3 drops of Lavender

How to Make It:

1) Add oils to a 10ml roller bottle and fill to the top with a carrier oil such as fractionated coconut oil. Shake bottle before each use.

2) Apply to the bottom of each foot or to wrists.

Note:

This recipe has a 3% dilution ratio. If you do not have bergamot try switching it out for cedarwood. You can adjust this recipe based on your needs, see the dilution chart on page 21. Recipe is meant for adults.

What You Need:

_____   _____

_____   _____

How to make It:

_____

_____

Note:

_____

_____

What You Need:

_____   _____

_____   _____

How to make It:

_____

_____

Note:

_____

_____

What You Need:

_____   _____

_____   _____

How to make It:

_____

_____

Note:

_____

_____

_____

What You Need:

_____   _____

_____   _____

How to make It:

_____

_____

Note:

_____

_____

What You Need:

_____   _____

_____   _____

How to make It:

_____

_____

Note:

_____

_____

_____

What You Need:

_____   _____

_____   _____

How to make It:

_____

_____

Note:

_____

_____

What You Need:

_____   _____

_____   _____

How to make It:

_____

_____

Note:

_____

_____

What You Need:

_____   _____

_____   _____

How to make It:

_____

_____

Note:

_____

_____

What You Need:

_____   _____

_____   _____

How to make It:

_____

_____

Note:

_____

_____

What You Need:

_____   _____

_____   _____

How to make It:

_____

_____

Note:

_____

_____

What You Need:

_____   _____

_____   _____

How to make It:

_____

_____

Note:

_____

_____

_____

What You Need:

_____   _____

_____   _____

How to make It:

_____

_____

Note:

_____

_____

What You Need:

_____   _____

_____   _____

How to make It:

_____

_____

Note:

_____

_____

What You Need:

_____   _____

_____   _____

How to make It:

_____

_____

Note:

_____

_____

What You Need:

_____   _____

_____   _____

How to make It:

_____

_____

Note:

_____

_____

_____

What You Need:

_____   _____

_____   _____

How to make It:

_____

_____

Note:

_____

_____

What You Need:

_____   _____

_____   _____

How to make It:

_____

_____

Note:

_____

_____

What You Need:

_____   _____

_____   _____

How to make It:

_____

_____

Note:

_____

_____

What You Need:

_____   _____

_____   _____

How to make It:

_____

_____

Note:

_____

_____

_____

What You Need:

_____   _____

_____   _____

How to make It:

_____

_____

Note:

_____

_____

What You Need:

_____   _____

_____   _____

How to make It:

_____

_____

Note:

_____

_____

_____

What You Need:

_____   _____

_____   _____

How to make It:

_____

_____

Note:

_____

_____

What You Need:

_____   _____

_____   _____

How to make It:

_____

_____

Note:

_____

_____

What You Need:

_____   _____

_____   _____

How to make It:

_____

_____

Note:

_____

_____

_____

What You Need:

_____   _____

_____   _____

How to make It:

_____

_____

Note:

_____

_____

_____

What You Need:

_____   _____

_____   _____

How to make It:

_____

_____

Note:

_____

_____

What You Need:

_____   _____

_____   _____

How to make It:

_____

_____

Note:

_____

_____

What You Need:

_____   _____

_____   _____

How to make It:

_____

_____

Note:

_____

_____

What You Need:

_____   _____

_____   _____

How to make It:

_____

_____

Note:

_____

_____

What You Need:

_____   _____

_____   _____

How to make It:

_____

_____

Note:

_____

_____

What You Need:

_____   _____

_____   _____

How to make It:

_____

_____

Note:

_____

_____

_____

What You Need:

_____   _____

_____   _____

How to make It:

_____

_____

Note:

_____

_____

Stop and Smell the Oils

Part 4: DIY Recipes

DIY Moisturizing Essential Oil Body Butter

What You Need:

1 cup of Shea Butter

½ cup of Olive Oil

½ cup of Coconut Oil

A glass container for storage

30 drops of Essential Oil (I used equal parts of lemon and lime)

How to Make It:

1) melt the shea butter, coconut oil and olive oil together in a pot on the stove top. Set to low/medium heat.

2) Once the ingredients have melted to a liquid, remove from heat and allow to cool until partly set. I transferred the liquid into a bowl and put it in the freezer for 20 minutes.

3) Add the essential oils to the bowl

4) Use a hand mixer and whip the ingredients for about 3 minutes until the body butter comes close to the consistency of butter cream frosting.

5) Place in a glass jar and use as you wish!

Note:

This body butter takes a while to absorb into your skin and you definitely do not want to apply it before putting your clothes on as I would imagine the oil could stain your clothes.

DIY All Natural Essential Oil Foaming Hand Soap

What You Need:

2 Tablespoons of Dr. Bronner's Castile Soap

1 1/2 Tablespoons of grapeseed oil or fractionated coconut oil

12 drops of essential oil (I used eucalyptus)

1 1/2 cups of water

A recycled foaming hand soap bottle

How to Make It:

1) Rinse and clean your recycled foaming hand soap bottle.

2) Add the soap, carrier oil and essential oil

3) Add the water to the bottle.

4) Screw the pump top on to the bottle and you are ready to use!

Helpful Tips:

Do not shake the bottle once you add the water. You will notice that the soap interacts with the water as soon as it is added and shaking could cause the bottle to overflow with soap suds.

You can choose any essential oil you would like, in fact you don't have to use any at all! I would not recommend using citrus oils as they can break down the plastic which could cause problems with how your pump works.

Essential Oil Sugar Scrub

What You Need:

I cup of white sugar

1/4 cup of a carrier oil of your choice (I used grapeseed oil)

6 drops of the essential oil of your choice (I used lime)

A glass jar for storage

How to Make It:

1) Pour the sugar into a mixing bowl. Break down any sugar clumps with a spoon.

2) Add the oil and essential oil of your choice to the sugar.

3) Fold the ingredients together until it is well mixed.

4) Pour the mixture into a glass jar for storage until you are ready to use it!

Note:

Lavender Essential Oil Play Dough

What You Need:

I cup of all purpose flour

1/2 cup of salt

I TBSP of cream of tartar

10-12 drops Lavender (or the oil of your choice)

I TBSP of olive oil

1 1/2 cups of boiling water

Food colouring (optional)

How to Make It:

1) Combine the flour, salt, and cream of tartar in a bowl and mix.

2) Add the olive oil and essential oils to the dry mixture (don't stir yet).

3) Measure out the boiling water. If you choose to use food colouring, mix it into the water while it is in the measuring cup.

4) Gradually pour the water into the mixture and stir until ingredients are mostly combined.

5) Knead the dough with your hands to make sure everything is combined but be sure to test the temperature of the dough first. If it is too hot, wait for it to cool down. Knead the dough until it is no longer sticky.

6) Let the dough cool and then you can play with it! Store in a zipped bag or sealed container to help it last longer between uses.

Homemade Relaxing Soap with Essential Oils

What You Need:

6oz of Shea Butter Soap Base

1 ½ teaspoons of oats

7 drops Lavender

7 drops Cedarwood

Silicone soap mold

How to Make It:

1) Cut the 6 oz of shea butter soap base into cubes.

2) Put the cubes into a glass bowl or glass measuring cup and put in the microwave for 30 seconds. Stir the soap base (which should be mostly liquid at this point) and put it back the microwave for another 15-20 seconds until all of the soap base has melted.

3) Add 1-½ teaspoons of oats to your soap base.

4) Add 7 drops of lavender and 7 drops of cedarwood essential oil.

5) Stir everything together.

6) Pour the mixture into your silicone mold.

7) Let sit for 2 hours

8) Pop the bars out of the mold and that's it, they are ready to use!

Note:

The yield will depend on the size of your soap mold. My mold allowed me to make 3 square bars.

What You Need:

_____   _____
_____   _____
_____   _____

How to Make It:

_____
_____
_____
_____
_____
_____
_____
_____
_____
_____
_____

Note:

_____
_____
_____

What You Need:

_____ _____

_____ _____

_____ _____

How to make It:

_____

_____

_____

_____

_____

_____

_____

_____

_____

_____

Note:

_____

_____

_____

What You Need:

_____   _____

_____   _____

_____   _____

How to make It:

_____

_____

_____

_____

_____

_____

_____

_____

_____

_____

_____

Note:

_____

_____

_____

What You Need:

_____   _____

_____   _____

_____   _____

How to make It:

_____

_____

_____

_____

_____

_____

_____

_____

_____

_____

Note:

_____

_____

_____

What You Need:

_____   _____

_____   _____

_____   _____

How to make It:

_____

_____

_____

_____

_____

_____

_____

_____

_____

_____

_____

Note:

_____

_____

_____

What You Need:

_____   _____

_____   _____

_____   _____

How to make It:

_____

_____

_____

_____

_____

_____

_____

_____

_____

_____

Note:

_____

_____

_____

What You Need:

_____   _____

_____   _____

_____   _____

How to make It:

_____

_____

_____

_____

_____

_____

_____

_____

_____

_____

Note:

_____

_____

_____

What You Need:

_____   _____

_____   _____

_____   _____

How to make It:

_____

_____

_____

_____

_____

_____

_____

_____

_____

_____

_____

Note:

_____

_____

_____

What You Need:

_____   _____

_____   _____

_____   _____

How to Make It:

_____

_____

_____

_____

_____

_____

_____

_____

_____

Note:

_____

_____

_____

What You Need:

_____   _____

_____   _____

_____   _____

How to make It:

_____

_____

_____

_____

_____

_____

_____

_____

_____

_____

_____

Note:

_____

_____

_____

What You Need:

_____   _____

_____   _____

_____   _____

How to make It:

_____

_____

_____

_____

_____

_____

_____

_____

_____

_____

Note:

_____

_____

_____

What You Need:

_____ _____

_____ _____

_____ _____

How to make It:

_____

_____

_____

_____

_____

_____

_____

_____

_____

_____

Note:

_____

_____

_____

What You Need:

_____   _____

_____   _____

_____   _____

How to make It:

_____

_____

_____

_____

_____

_____

_____

_____

_____

_____

Note:

_____

_____

_____

What You Need:

_____   _____

_____   _____

_____   _____

How to make It:

_____

_____

_____

_____

_____

_____

_____

_____

_____

_____

_____

Note:

_____

_____

_____

What You Need:

_____   _____

_____   _____

_____   _____

How to Make It:

_____

_____

_____

_____

_____

_____

_____

_____

_____

_____

Note:

_____

_____

_____

What You Need:

_____   _____

_____   _____

_____   _____

How to make It:

_____

_____

_____

_____

_____

_____

_____

_____

_____

_____

Note:

_____

_____

_____

What You Need:

_____   _____

_____   _____

_____   _____

How to make It:

_____

_____

_____

_____

_____

_____

_____

_____

_____

_____

Note:

_____

_____

_____

What You Need:

_____ _____

_____ _____

_____ _____

How to make It:

_____

_____

_____

_____

_____

_____

_____

_____

_____

_____

Note:

_____

_____

_____

What You Need:

_____   _____

_____   _____

_____   _____

How to make It:

_____

_____

_____

_____

_____

_____

_____

_____

_____

Note:

_____

_____

_____

What You Need:

_____   _____

_____   _____

_____   _____

How to make It:

_____

_____

_____

_____

_____

_____

_____

_____

_____

_____

Note:

_____

_____

_____

What You Need:

_____   _____

_____   _____

_____   _____

How to make It:

_____

_____

_____

_____

_____

_____

_____

_____

_____

_____

_____

Note:

_____

_____

_____

There is oil
in the house
of the wise.

Proverbs 21:20

Part 5: Cleaning Recipes

All-Natural Toilet Bowl Cleaning Pods

What You Need:

½ cup of Citric Acid

1 cup of Baking Soda

2 Tbsp of water

20 drops Lemon OR Orange

Silicone mold

2 mixing Bowls

10 drops Tea Tree OR Eucalyptus

How to Make It:

1) It is important that you follow these directions in these specific steps as the citric acid with react with liquid so you want to make sure you add it slowly and as described below.

In Bowl 1 (liquids):

2) mix 2 Tbsp of water with 30 drops of essential oil

In Bowl 2 (solids):

3) mix ½ cup of citric acid and 1 cup of baking soda

Combining Ingredients:

4) Slowly add a portion of bowl 1 (liquid) into bowl 2 (solids).

5) Repeat steps 1 & 2 until the mixture somewhat solidifies. The best way to test this is to scoop some into the palm of your hand, gently squeeze it and see if it holds its shape.

6) Now press the mixture into your silicone mold. Be sure to pack it into the mold.

7) Stir the liquid into the solids.

8) Let the pods sit in the mold overnight.

9) You are now ready to use your all natural toilet bowl cleaning pods! Drop the pod in the toilet, let it fizz around, give it a quick scrub and you're done!

10) Put the remaining pods in an airtight container and store in a cool place away from moisture (so the pods don't activate).

Note:

_____

_____

_____

Disinfecting Bathroom Cleaning Spray

What You Need:

A glass or aluminum spray bottle

1 cup Water

1/2 cup White Vinegar

8 drops Lemon

8 drops Tea Tree

6 drops White Fir

How to Make It:

1) Combine all ingredients in your spray bottle make sure to shake the bottle before use as the oils will settle to the top after being stored.

2) Get to cleaning!

Note:

Adjust recipe in order to make smaller/larger batches.

What You Need:

_____   _____

_____   _____

_____   _____

How to make It:

_____

_____

_____

_____

_____

_____

_____

_____

_____

_____

Note:

_____

_____

_____

What You Need:

_____ _____

_____ _____

_____ _____

How to make It:

_____

_____

_____

_____

_____

_____

_____

_____

_____

_____

Note:

_____

_____

_____

What You Need:

_____   _____

_____   _____

_____   _____

How to make It:

_____

_____

_____

_____

_____

_____

_____

_____

_____

_____

Note:

_____

_____

_____

_____

What You Need:

_____   _____

_____   _____

_____   _____

How to make It:

_____

_____

_____

_____

_____

_____

_____

_____

_____

Note:

_____

_____

_____

What You Need:

_____   _____

_____   _____

_____   _____

How to make It:

_____

_____

_____

_____

_____

_____

_____

_____

_____

_____

Note:

_____

_____

_____

What You Need:

_____   _____

_____   _____

_____   _____

How to make It:

_____

_____

_____

_____

_____

_____

_____

_____

_____

_____

_____

Note:

_____

_____

_____

What You Need:

_____   _____

_____   _____

_____   _____

How to make It:

_____

_____

_____

_____

_____

_____

_____

_____

_____

_____

Note:

_____

_____

_____

What You Need:

_____   _____

_____   _____

_____   _____

How to make It:

_____

_____

_____

_____

_____

_____

_____

_____

_____

_____

Note:

_____

_____

_____

What You Need:

_____   _____

_____   _____

_____   _____

How to make It:

_____

_____

_____

_____

_____

_____

_____

_____

_____

_____

_____

Note:

_____

_____

_____

What You Need:

_____   _____

_____   _____

_____   _____

How to make It:

_____

_____

_____

_____

_____

_____

_____

_____

_____

_____

Note:

_____

_____

_____

What You Need:

_____   _____

_____   _____

_____   _____

How to Make It:

_____

_____

_____

_____

_____

_____

_____

_____

_____

_____

_____

Note:

_____

_____

_____

What You Need:

_____   _____

_____   _____

_____   _____

How to make It:

_____

_____

_____

_____

_____

_____

_____

_____

_____

_____

Note:

_____

_____

_____

Well, that's a wrap! Thank you so much for purchasing this book, I hope you find it helpful in keeping your essential oil recipes organized!

If you are looking for great places to find essential oil recipes check out my blog at www.paintedteacup.com where you will find links to both my Facebook and Pinterest profiles. I love sharing and posting new recipes all the time.

Remember when looking at recipes to consider the dilution ratio. If you feel that there are too many drops of oil used in the recipe, simply reduce the drops. Also when looking for recipes for kids please be cautious of the oils used. There are many people who use the oils listed 'don't use' with their children so if you are considering using them I would recommend that you do your research first.

More Publications:
If you want to read more by Painted Teacup you can purchase *"Essential Oils Made Easy: DIY Diffuser & Roller Bottle Recipes"* on Amazon.

Helpful Resources:
Essential Oil Safety Textbook by Robert Tisserand & Rodney Young this book can be purchased as a physical book, an ebook, or you can even 'rent' a copy on Amazon! Alternatively you can check out www.roberttisserand.com to read the blog posts he has written.

Dilution Calculator: Head over to marvymoms.com where they have a cool calculator that helps you to determine the dilution percentages. There are 2 features depending on what you need. One let's you enter the dilution percentage you are trying to achieve and it will tell you how many drops you need based on the container size you entered. Or in the other section you can enter the size of bottle and number of drops used and it will give you the dilution percentage of the recipe you have.

Chantal and April's Journey began many years ago in a small town in Southwestern Ontario. Luckily, both of their parents knew their distaste for early mornings and they were enrolled in the afternoon class of Junior Kindergarten. From that first day of school till 20 something years later they have been inseparable. They are once again combining their varied and innumerable talents to bring you the *Essential Oil Toolkit & Recipe Journal*.

Author

Chantal Bernard of Painted Teacup

Chantal is a full time blogger and virtual assistant with a background in social work. Chantal is the face behind paintedteacup.com where she shares information & support in the areas of essential oils, mental health & chronic illness. When not working on the blog or doing client work Chantal enjoys spending time with her husband & their little chihuahua Tikka.

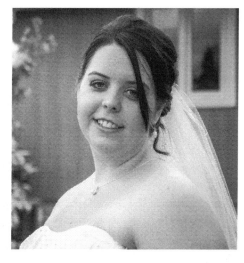

Chantal's journey with essential oils started in 2014 when her grandmother wanted to share oils with her when she was feeling under the weather. She was skeptical at first, but quickly realized that the oils helped. Since then essential oils are a prominent part of Chantal's daily routine. Chantal has had a wonderful experience using essential oils and is passionate about sharing knowledge, support and resources to encourage others in their essential oil journey.

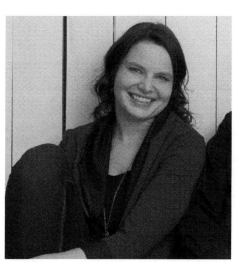

Designer

April Berry of Wildberry Designs

April is a Marketing Coordinator by day and a freelance designer by night. Wildberry Designs was started in 2016 after April realized her passion for design and creating beautiful layouts for books and electronic artwork. She loves learning and is always looking for a new challenge! You can check out more of her work at www.wildberrydesigns.ca

April lives in London, ON with her partner and their two beautiful dogs, Dakota and Luca.

Notes

Notes

Notes

Notes

Notes

Notes

Notes

Notes

Index

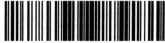

Made in the USA
San Bernardino, CA
08 May 2018